Table of Contents

PREVIEW 4

PANCREATIC CANCER DIET RECIPES 7

BREAKFAST 7

1. Keto Chicken and Waffles (Low Carb) 7

2. Chicken and Waffles... 10

3. Chicken Paprikash... 13

4. Chicken Lo Mein.. 15

5. Keto Sesame Chicken (Low Carb) 17

6. Keto Chicken Fajita Casserole (Low Carb Bake).................... 19

7. Easy Chicken Cordon Bleu 21

8. Chicken Alfredo and Shrimp (Fettuccine Alfredo)................. 23

9. Orange Chicken... 26

10. Keto Chinese Chicken and Broccoli (Low Carb) 29

LUNCH... 31

11. Keto Chicken and Asparagus (One Skillet)......................... 31

12. Keto Chicken Fajita Soup (Crockpot, Instant Pot & Stovetop)

.... 33

13. Keto Jalapeno Popper Chicken Casserole (Low Carb) 36

14. Keto Chicken Noodle Soup (Low Carb5 38

15. Keto Buffalo Chicken Casserole (Low Carb) 41

16. Keto Thai Coconut Chicken Soup (Low Carb) 43

17. Keto Chicken Caesar Salad {Low Carb} 45

18. Keto Grilled Chicken Thighs (Low Carb) 48

19. Keto Pulled Chicken (Slow Cooker or Instant Pot) 50

20. Keto Coconut Chicken (Low Carb Curry) 53

DINNER 55

21. Keto Chicken Fried Rice Cauliflower (Low Carb) 55

22. Keto Avocado Chicken Salad (Low Carb) 57

23. Easy Chicken Casserole 58

24. Blackened Chicken 60

25. Keto Chinese Chicken and Broccoli (Low Carb) 62

26. Keto Balsamic Caprese Chicken (Low Carb) 64

27. Keto Slow Cooker Ranch Chicken (Low Carb) 66

28. Baked Chicken 67

29. Chicken Marsala 69

30. Chicken Stew 71

PREVIEW

Pancreatic cancer occurs when cells in your pancreas mutate (change) and multiply out of control, forming a tumor. Your pancreas is a gland in your abdomen (belly), between your spine and stomach. It makes hormones that control blood-sugar levels and enzymes that aid in digestion.

Most pancreatic cancers start in the ducts of your pancreas. The main pancreatic duct (the duct of Wirsung) connects your pancreas to your common bile duct.

Early-stage pancreatic tumors don't show up on imaging tests. For this reason, many people don't receive a diagnosis until the cancer has spread (metastasis). Pancreatic cancer is also resistant to many common cancer drugs, making it notoriously difficult to treat.

Ongoing research focuses on early detection through genetic testing and new imaging methods. Still, there's much to learn.

The pancreas secretes enzymes that aid digestion and hormones that help regulate the metabolism of sugars. This type of cancer is often detected late, spreads rapidly and has a poor prognosis.

There are no symptoms in the early stages. Later stages are associated with symptoms, but these can be non-specific, such as lack of appetite and weight loss.

Treatment may include surgically removing the pancreas, radiation and chemotherapy.

Pancreatic cancer is responsible for approximately 3% of all cancers in the United States. Its the 10th most common cancer in men and people assigned male at birth, and the 8th most common cancer in women and people assigned female at birth.

Pancreatic tumors are either exocrine or neuroendocrine (endocrine) tumors. This is based on the type of cell they start in. Knowing the type of tumor is important because each type acts differently and responds to different treatments.

More than 90% of pancreatic cancers are exocrine tumors. The most common type of pancreatic cancer is adenocarcinoma.

Less than 10% of pancreatic tumors are neuroendocrine tumors (pancreatic NETs or PNETs), also called islet cell tumors. They often grow slower than exocrine tumors.

Changes in your DNA cause cancer. These can be inherited from your parents or can arise over time. The changes that arise over time can happen because you were exposed to something harmful. They can also happen randomly.

Pancreatic cancer's exact causes are not well understood. About 10% of pancreatic cancers are considered familial or hereditary. Most pancreatic cancer happens randomly or is caused by things such as smoking, obesity and age.

If you are a first-degree relative of someone diagnosed with pancreatic cancer, you may have an increased risk of developing pancreatic cancer. Your family member with pancreatic cancer is strongly recommended to undergo genetic testing for inherited mutations.

PANCREATIC CANCER DIET RECIPES

BREAKFAST

1. Keto Chicken and Waffles (Low Carb)

Prep Time: 20 Minutes

Cook Time: 30 Minutes

Servings: 8

Ingredients

For the Waffles:

- 2 cups almond flour, blanched
- 1 tsp baking powder
- 1/2 tsp salt
- 1 tablespoon erythritol
- 1 teaspoon vanilla
- 1 cup heavy whipping cream (or buttermilk)
- 4 tbsp butter melted
- 4 large eggs

For the chicken:

- 2 pound boneless, skinless chicken breast cut into tender pieces

- 3/4 cup almond flour, blanched
- 1 teaspoon onion powder
- 1 large egg
- 1 tbsp paprika
- 1 tsp garlic powder
- Salt and pepper to taste

For Topping:

- Sugar Free Syrup
- Tools
- Parchment paper
- Baking Sheet
- Waffle maker

Instructions

For the waffles:

1. Preheat the waffle maker on high heat.
2. Whisk together baking powder, flour, and salt in a bowl and whisk eggs, cream, and other ingredients on the other bowl.
3. Add the wet mixture into the dry and stir until combined.

4. Lightly grease the waffle maker with non-stick cooking spray.

5. Pour 1/2 cup of batter and cook for 5 minutes or until steam coming from waffle maker stops or slows down a bit.

6. Open the waffle maker and remove waffle and repeat the same process for the remaining batter, regreasing the iron in between.

7. Done!

For the chicken:

1. Preheat the oven to 425 F, and line a baking sheet with parchment paper.

2. In a shallow bowl, combine the almond flour with the seasonings and beat the eggs into another bowl.

3. Toss the chicken pieces into the almond seasoning mixture, then dip it into the egg mixture and single layer them on the baking sheet.

4. Place the chicken in the oven and bake for 10-12 minutes or until chicken is crispy and cooked through, flipping once halfway through.

5. Serve the waffles topped with chicken and drizzle with your favorite sugar-free syrup.

2. Chicken and Waffles

Prep Time: 20 Minutes

Cook Time: 10 Minutes

Servings: 4

Ingredients

- 8 chicken tenders
- 2 cups buttermilk
- 1 teaspoon garlic salt
- 1 tablespoon onion powder
- 2 teaspoons Worcestershire
- 2 teaspoons paprika
- 4 tablespoons cornstarch
- 2 teaspoons hot sauce
- 2 teaspoons black pepper
- 3 tablespoons seasoned salt
- 2 1/2 cups all-purpose flour

Instructions

1. In a medium bowl, whisk together hot sauce, buttermilk, and Worcestershire sauce and pour

mixture over chicken pieces to a ziploc bag or an airtight container.

2. Let it marinate in the refrigerator up to 8 hours or at least 2 hours if you are in hurry.

3. Meanwhile, Toast waffles according to package instructions.

4. In a separate bowl, add cornstarch, flour, paprika, black pepper, seasoned salt, garlic salt, and onion powder and mix all together.

5. Once you are finished with the marinating, add some marinade from the chicken to your flour mixture to form crumbs.

6. Now remove chicken from marinade and put it into the flour mixture (Flour crumbs) to coat the chicken.

7. In a skillet, heat oil over medium-high heat (275 degrees)

8. Now fry all the coated chicken pieces, four pieces at a time, and fry until crispy and golden brown on both sides.

9. Remove the chicken and place on paper towel sheet covered with parchment to drain.

10. Lightly warm the waffles and add butter and allow to melt.

11. Layer each waffle with two chicken pieces, drizzle with pure maple syrup or syrup of your own choice.

12. Serve immediately.

3. Chicken Paprikash

Prep Time: 5 Minutes

Cook Time: 45 Minutes

Servings: 6

Ingredients

- 2 Pounds chicken thighs, with skin
- 2 Tbsp. extra-virgin olive oil
- 1 large onion, chopped
- Kosher salt
- Freshly ground black pepper
- 2 Tbsp. all-purpose flour
- 1 (28-oz.) can crushed tomatoes
- 3 cloves garlic, minced
- 1 Cup low-sodium chicken broth
- 12 Ounces egg noodles, cooked according to package directions
- 1/2 Cup sour cream
- 3 tbsp. paprika
- Freshly chopped parsley, for garnish

Instructions

1. Preheat oven to 400°F. Season both sides of chicken with salt and pepper. Heat oil in a large skillet over medium heat.
2. Add chicken and cook for 8 minutes per side until skin is golden and cooked through. Remove chicken pieces from skillet (reserve fat in the pan).
3. Add onion and garlic and saute for 5 minutes, until soft and fragrant.
4. Add flour and paprika and cook for 1 minuter.
5. Now add chicken broth and crushed tomatoes and stir until combined.
6. Return chicken to the pan and cook for 20 minutes until chicken is cooked through and the bones fall apart.
7. Turn off the heat and stir in sour cream.
8. Serve over Rice or egg noodles and garnish with parsley.

4. Chicken Lo Mein

Prep Time: 10 Minutes

Cook Time: 25 Minutes

Servings: 4

Ingredients

- 8 ounce lo mein noodles
- 1 Lb boneless skinless chicken breast, cut into 1" pieces
- 1 head broccoli, cut into small florets
- 1 red bell pepper, chopped
- 1 tbsp. canola oil
- 1 teaspoon sesame oil
- 1/4 cup hoisin sauce
- 1 cup snow peas
- 1 cup carrot, peeled and grated
- 1/4 cup low-sodium soy sauce

Instructions

1. Cook noodles according to package instructions. Drain and toss with sesame oil to coat.

2. In a large skillet add canola oil over medium-high heat. Add bell pepper and broccoli and cook for 6-7 minutes until tender.
3. Stir in chicken and cook for 8 minutes until golden and no longer pink from inside.
4. Add cooked noodles, carrots, hoisin sauce, snow peas, and soy sauce and toss all together.
5. Serve!

5. Keto Sesame Chicken (Low Carb)

Prep Time: 15 Minutes

Cook Time: 15 Minutes

Servings: 3

Ingredients

For the chicken:

- 1 pound chicken thighs, cut into bite sized pieces
- 1 egg, large
- 1 tbsp corn starch (or arrowroot powder)
- 1 tbsp sesame oil, toasted
- Salt and pepper

For the sauce:

- 2 tbsp coconut aminos (or gluten free soy sauce)
- 1 tbsp sesame oil, toasted
- 2 tbsp Sukrin Gold or lakanto golden monkfruit sweetener
- 1 tbsp vinegar, distilled
- 1 tsp ginger, freshly grated
- 1 clove garlic, minced
- 2 tbsp sesame seeds

- 1/4 tsp xanthan gum

Instructions

1. Take a bowl, beat the egg and add a tablespoon of arrowroot powder, mix well to make a batter.
2. Add in chicken thigh pieces and coat them well.
3. Heat a large pan, add a tablespoon of oil and once hot, add the chicken thighs one by one to avoid sticking to each other.
4. Fry the chicken for about 10 minutes or until golden brown on both sides.
5. Meanwhile, combine all the sauce ingredients in a bowl to make the sauce.
6. When the chicken is cooked through, pour the sauce directly to the pan and stir to combine. Reduce the heat and cook for 5 minutes or until the sauce has reached your desired thickness.
7. Done! Take out from the pan, sprinkle with scallions and sesame seeds on the top and serve over cauliflower rice or broccoli.

6. Keto Chicken Fajita Casserole (Low Carb Bake)

Prep Time: 10 Minutes

Cook Time: 50 Minutes

Servings: 12

Ingredients

- 3 chicken breast, boneless, skinless
- 2 tablespoons taco seasoning, divided
- 1/4 cup canned Rotel diced tomatoes and green chilies
- 1 red bell pepper, thinly sliced (seeds removed)
- 1 green bell pepper, thinly sliced (seeds removed)
- 1 medium onion, sliced
- 1/2 cup cheddar cheese, shredded
- 1/2 cup Monterrey jack cheese, shredded
- 8 ounces cream cheese, softened
- 1/4 cup heavy cream

Instructions

1. Preheat oven to 350 degrees.
2. In a baking tray, place the chicken, season with salt and pepper, and bake for about 20 - 25 minutes until no

longer pink. You can also use leftover rotisserie chicken or turkey.

3. Remove the chicken from the oven, and let it completely cool.
4. Heat a skillet over medium heat. Add bell peppers, onion, and Rotel canned tomatoes. Saute until vegetables are tender. Transfer to a bowl and set aside.
5. Chop the chicken into bite-sized chunks or thinly slice them lengthwise, and then add it to the vegetable bowl.
6. Add 1 tbsp. of taco seasoning and mix it together.
7. Now add half of the shredded cheese and the heavy cream to the bowl. Mix until combined. Add the remaining taco seasoning and stir everything until well combined.
8. Arrange the chicken mixture into a casserole dish (13.25"x8.5"), top with the remaining shredded cheese.
9. Place in the oven and bake for about 30 - 35 minutes until hot and bubbly.

7. Easy Chicken Cordon Bleu

Prep Time: 10 Minutes

Cook Time: 35 Minutes

Servings: 4

Ingredients

- 4 skinless, boneless chicken breast halves
- 6 slices Swiss cheese
- 1/4 teaspoon salt
- 1/2 cup seasoned bread crumbs
- 4 slices cooked ham
- 1/8 teaspoon ground black pepper

Instructions

1. Preheat oven to 175 degrees C (350 degrees F). With nonstick cooking spray coat your baking dish.
2. Pound chicken breasts to 1/4 inch thickness.
3. Sprinkle each piece of chicken with salt and pepper on both sides. Place 1 ham slice & cheese on top of each breast. Roll up each breast, and secure with a toothpick.

4. Sprinkle chicken with bread crumbs until fully covered.

5. Bake for 30 to 35 minutes, until chicken is no longer pink and juices run clear.

6. Place 1/2 cheese slice on top of each breast and return to oven cook until cheese has melted for 3 to 5 minutes. Remove toothpicks, and serve immediately.

8. Chicken Alfredo and Shrimp (Fettuccine Alfredo)

Prep Time: 10 Minutes

Cook Time: 30 Minutes

Servings: 5

Ingredients

- 1 chicken breast, skinless, boneless, cut into 1-inch cubes
- 3/4 pound medium/large shrimp (about 16), peeled and deveined, tails removed (if frozen, thawed)
- 12 oz. fettuccine
- 1/2 cup butter, unsalted (about 8 tbsp)
- 2 cups heavy cream (or half and half)
- 1 1/2 cups Parmigiano-Reggiano cheese, freshly grated (or grated Romano cheese)
- 1/2 - 1 tbsp cajun seasoning
- Freshly ground black pepper, to taste
- Kosher salt
- 2 pinches nutmeg, freshly grated
- 2 tbsp olive oil, for cooking and tossing

1. Heat a large pot, add water and salt, and bring it to a boil.
2. Add pasta, and cook as per the package instruction until tender or al dente but still slightly firm.
3. Strain, and toss with little olive oil to avoid sticking.
4. Pat dry the shrimp with a paper towel, season with salt and pepper.
5. Season the chicken with cajun seasoning, salt, and pepper.
6. Heat a large skillet over medium heat, add 2 tbsp of the butter, once melted, add the shrimp, raise the heat to medium-high and cook for about 3-4 minutes or until cooked through, flipping them in between. Transfer to a bowl and set aside.
7. On the same pan, add olive oil or butter. Add the chicken and cook for about 5-8 minutes or until no longer pink from inside and cooked through. Set aside.
8. Reduce the heat to medium, add the remaining butter. Scrape off any bits sticking to the bottom of the skillet with a wooden spoon. When the butter has fully melted, whisk in the cream and nutmeg and bring it to a simmer, lower the heat and cook for 2-3 minutes.

9. Whisk in Parmigiano cheese into the sauce. Add the cooked shrimp, chicken and pasta, toss well to combine.

10. Season with salt and pepper. Garnish with bacon bits and serve hot.

9. Orange Chicken

Prep Time: 40 Minutes

Cook Time: 40 Minutes

Servings: 4

Ingredients

For Sauce

- 1/3 cup rice vinegar
- 2 1/2 tablespoons soy sauce
- 1 1/2 cups water
- 2 tablespoons orange juice
- 1/4 cup lemon juice
- 1/2 teaspoon minced fresh ginger root
- 1/2 teaspoon minced garlic
- 1 tablespoon grated orange zest
- 1 cup packed brown sugar
- 1/4 teaspoon red pepper flakes
- 3 tablespoons cornstarch
- 2 tablespoons chopped green onion
- 2 tablespoons water

For Chicken

- 1/4 teaspoon salt
- 1/4 teaspoon pepper
- 2 boneless, skinless chicken breasts, cut into 1/2 inch pieces
- 1 cup all-purpose flour
- 3 tablespoons olive oil
- Toasted sesame seeds

Instructions

1. Set your saucepan over medium-high heat and pour orange juice, lemon juice, rice vinegar, 1 1/2 cups water, and soy sauce. Stir in the orange zest, ginger, garlic, brown sugar, chopped onion, and red pepper flakes. Bring to a boil and then cool down for 10 to 15 minutes.
2. Now pour 1 cup of sauce over the chicken pieces and refrigerate at least 2 hours.
3. In another bowl, mix the salt, flour, and pepper and add the marinated chicken pieces to coat.
4. In a large skillet heat the olive oil over medium heat and brown the chicken pieces on both sides. Drain on a plate lined with paper towels.

5. Now add sauce to the the skillet over medium-high heat and bring to a boil. Prepare a cornstarch mixture by mixing together the cornstarch and 2 tablespoons water and stir into the sauce. Add the chicken pieces, and simmer, about 5 minutes, stirring occasionally.

6. Heat the sesame seeds in a frying pan over medium heat about 30 seconds shaking the pan frequently.

7. Garnish with sesame seeds and serve with cauliflower rice or steamed rice.

10. Keto Chinese Chicken and Broccoli (Low Carb)

Prep Time: 10 Minutes

Cook Time: 20 Minutes

Servings: 4

Ingredients

- 1 lb chicken breasts, boneless skinless, cut into strips
- 2 cups broccoli florets, raw
- 1 tablespoon olive oil
- ½ teaspoon sesame oil
- ½ cup liquid aminos (or low carb soy sauce)
- ¼ cup chicken broth
- 3 tablespoon Swerve brown sugar substitute
- 1 teaspoon ginger paste
- 3 teaspoon garlic, minced
- ¼ teaspoon xanthan gum, optional
- 1 tablespoon sesame seeds

Instructions

1. Heat a skillet over medium-high heat. Add sesame and olive oil.

2. Add the chicken, and cook for 3-5 minutes on each side until browned and cooked through. Remove the chicken and set aside.

3. Reduce the heat to medium, add the broccoli florets, place on the lid, and cook until the broccoli is halfway cooked.

4. Add the chicken back to the skillet. Stir well.

5. In a mixing bowl, add the brown sugar substitute, soy sauce, chicken broth, minced garlic, and garlic paste. Combine well.

6. Pour the sauce mixture into the skillet over the chicken and broccoli. Toss to coat.

7. Add xanthan gum to thicken the sauce as per your liking. Add a little at a time. Add more liquid if it's too thick.

8. Let it cook for a few more minutes or until the chicken and broccoli have soaked enough sauce flavors. Sprinkle with sesame seeds.

LUNCH

11. Keto Chicken and Asparagus (One Skillet)

Prep Time: 5 Minutes

Cook Time: 20 Minutes

Servings: 4

Ingredients

- 4 chicken breasts, boneless, skinless, cut into thin cutlets
- 1/2 tsp garlic powder
- 2 Tbsp butter
- 2 Tbsp olive oil
- 1 shallot, minced (or sliced medium onion)
- 12 stalks fresh asparagus, ends trimmed and cut into 3-inch
- 1 cup heavy cream (or half and half)
- 1 tbsp fresh parsley, chopped
- Salt and pepper, or to taste

Instructions

1. Pound the chicken on all sides. Season the cutlets with salt, pepper, and garlic powder.

2. Heat a large skillet over medium high heat. Add olive oil, once hot, add the chicken breasts and cook uncovered for about 3 to 4 minutes on each side or until golden brown. Remove from the skillet and set aside.

3. Add the butter to the skillet. Add trimmed asparagus, salt, and pepper. Stir cook for 2-3 minutes. Add minced shallot, cover, and cook for about 3 minutes, string occasionally or until tender and crisp.

4. Add the heavy cream, increase the heat to medium-high, bring to a simmer, and let cook for 3-4 minutes, stirring often.

5. Add extra with salt and pepper as per your taste.

6. Place the butter fried chicken in the skillet over the creamy asparagus and spoon some sauce over the chicken.

7. Sprinkle fresh chopped parsley and serve hot.

12. Keto Chicken Fajita Soup (Crockpot, Instant Pot & Stovetop)

Prep Time: 5 Minutes

Cook Time: 25 Minutes

Servings: 6

Ingredients

- 1.5 pound chicken breasts, boneless, skinless
- 2 tablespoons ghee (or butter)
- 1 green bell pepper, chopped
- 1(14.5 ounces) can diced tomatoes, drained (fire-roasted)
- 1 red bell pepper, chopped
- 1/2 white onion, chopped
- 3 minced garlic cloves
- 1 limc, juiced
- 8 oz cream cheese
- 4 cups chicken stock (or broth)
- 2 tbsp of Fajita seasoning (or homemade)

Instructions

Instant Pot

1. Turn on the instant pot to saute mode. Add ghee, once hot, add peppers, onion, and garlic. Stir cook for 1-2 minutes
2. Turn off the saute feature. Add the chicken breasts (whole), chicken broth, drained canned tomatoes, and fajita seasoning to the pot. Secure the lid, turn to seal, and set the time for 5 minutes on high pressure.
3. Do a quick pressure release? Open the lid, shred the chicken using 2 forks.
4. Stir in the cream cheese and lime juice, stir until well incorporated into the soup.
5. Turn on the saute mode if the cheese is not melting well.
6. Serve immediately with a lime slice, sliced avocado, guacamole, sour cream, and shredded cheese.

Crockpot

1. Dump everything into the pot (6qt Crockpot) except cream cheese and lime juice.
2. Cook on low for 6-7 hours or on high for 3-4 hours.

3. Once cooked, remove chicken, shred and put it back to the Crockpot. Stir in cream cheese and lime juice and let cook until cheese is melted.

4. Serve immediately.

Stovetop

1. Cook and shred the chicken.

2. Heat a large pot over medium-high heat. Add ghee, once hot, add garlic, onion, and peppers. Cook for 1-2 minutes.

3. Reduce the heat to low and pour in chicken broth, canned tomatoes, seasoning, and cream cheese in the pot, whisk until well incorporated.

4. Add in shredded chicken and give it a good stir and let it cook until the cream cheese has completely melted.

5. Serve immediately and enjoy!

13. Keto Jalapeno Popper Chicken Casserole (Low Carb)

Prep Time: 10 Minutes

Cook Time: 45 Minutes

Servings: 8

Ingredients

- 6 chicken breast, boneless, skinless
- Salt and pepper, to taste
- Jalapeno Popper Layer
- 1/4 cup jalapeno slices, diced
- 5 slices of bacon, diced
- 1/2 cup mayonnaise (or plain yogurt)
- 1 (8 oz) package cream cheese, softened
- 1 cup cheddar cheese, shredded
- 1/2 cup Kraft Parmesan, grated
- 1/4 cup onion, diced
- Topping
- 1/2 cup Kraft grated Parmesan Cheese
- 2 oz bag of crushed pork skins (chicharron)
- 4 tablespoon melted butter

Instructions

1. Preheat oven to 425 degrees.
2. In a 13×9 casserole dish, Place the chicken, season with salt and pepper, and bake for about 30-40 minutes.
3. Meanwhile, heat a skillet and fry the bacon pieces until crispy. Remove and add onions and saute until tender. Set aside.
4. In a mixing bowl, add fried crispy bacon, onions, mayonnaise, and cream cheese, cheddar, and Parmesan cheese. Combine well.
5. Remove the chicken and set the oven to 350 degrees.
6. Spread the cheese jalapeno pepper mixture evenly all over until each chicken breast is well covered.
7. Put in back to the oven and bake for 15 more minutes or until topping starts to brown and bubbly.
8. While it's cooking, mix the Parmesan cheese, crushed pork skins, and melted butter all together.
9. After 15 minutes, sprinkle the mixture on top of the popper chicken and then broil for a couple of minutes until pork skins are browned. Have a close look to not burn it.
10. Enjoy!

14. Keto Chicken Noodle Soup (Low Carb5

Prep Time: 10 Minutes

Cook Time: 30 Minutes

Servings: 4

Ingredients

Soup

- 2 cups shredded chicken, cooked
- 3 cups chicken bone broth
- 2 tablespoons butter
- ¼ cup chopped carrots
- 3 stalks celery, sliced
- ½ cup diced onion
- ½ teaspoon salt
- 1 bay leaf

Egg Noodles

- 1 egg
- 1 tablespoon xanthan gum
- 1 cup almond flour
- ½ teaspoon onion powder, optional
- ½ teaspoon salt

- ⅓ Cup water, luke warm

Instructions

1. Preheat oven to 200 degrees.
2. Heat a large stock pot over medium high heat. Add butter and let it melt. Add onion, carrots, celery, and salt. Cook until just tender (do not cook completely).
3. Pour in chicken broth, add bay leaf, shredded chicken. Stir everything, bring to a rolling boil, then reduce the heat and simmer uncovered.
4. Meanwhile, let's prepare the egg noodles, in a small mixing bowl, add almond flour, xanthan gum, salt, and onion powder (optional), and combine well.
5. Add egg with hot water. Whisk well until well combined and make a dought out of it.
6. Take two sheets of parchment paper and place the dough in between.
7. Roll the dough from over the parchment paper and then slice into ¼ inch thick using a pizza cutter or knife.
8. Lay a sheet of parchment paper into the baking tray, transfer the noodles and bake for about 15 to 20 minutes at 200 degrees.

9. After its done cooking, remove noodles from the oven.

10. Turn off the stovetop, add the noodles to the soup.

11. Serve hot immediately.

15. Keto Buffalo Chicken Casserole (Low Carb)

Prep Time: 15 Minutes

Cook Time: 30 Minutes

Servings: 4

Ingredients

- 2 cups chicken, cooked (use rotisserie chicken)
- 2 cloves garlic, crushed
- 1/2 cup hot sauce
- 2 cups cauliflower, chopped
- 3 tablespoons heavy cream
- 4 ounces cheddar cheese, grated
- 4 ounces cream cheese

Instructions

1. Preheat the oven to 400°F.
2. Put the cauliflower into the microwave for 4-5 minutes.
3. Meanwhile, in a skillet, add the hot sauce, cream cheese, garlic, and cook until cheese is melted. Add the chicken and cauliflower and give it a good mix until combined.

4. Lightly spray the baking dish with non-stick spray. Spread the mixture into the dish, then pour the heavy cream and sprinkle the cheddar cheese over the top.

5. Place the baking dish into the oven and bake for about 30-35 minutes until hot and bubbly and nicely browned on the top.

6. Remove from the oven, cool down a little bit, and enjoy.

16. Keto Thai Coconut Chicken Soup (Low Carb)

Prep Time: 5 Minutes

Cook Time: 30 Minutes

Servings: 6

Ingredients

- 4 chicken breasts, cut into bite-sized
- 14 oz chicken broth (or vegetable stock)
- ¼ cup red boat fish sauce
- 14 oz full fat coconut milk
- 2 tbsp Thai garlic chili paste
- 1 oz lime juice
- 1 tbsp coconut aminos (or liquid aminos)
- 2 sprigs Thai basil fresh (if not available, use dried basil)
- 1 tsp ground ginger
- Chopped cilantro, to garnish
- 3 1/2 water

Instructions

1. Heat a large stock pot over high heat, add water, chicken broth, lime juice, coconut milk, chili sauce, coconut aminos, fish sauce, ginger, and basil. Combine well and bring to a boil.

2. Reduce heat to low-medium, add in chicken pieces, stir well, cover with the lid and simmer for about 25-30 minutes.

3. After it's done, remove basil leaves and garnish with cilantro.

17. Keto Chicken Caesar Salad {Low Carb}

Prep Time: 15 Minutes

Cook Time: 15 Minutes

Servings: 4

Ingredients

For chicken:

- 4 Chicken Breasts, boneless, skinless
- 1/2 tsp. Kosher Salt
- 2 tbsp. Olive Oil
- 1 tbsp. Dried Oregano

For Salad:

- 4 boiled eggs, then peeled and quartered
- 1/4 cup grated Parmesan cheese
- 2 Avocado, medium size, pitted and chopped
- 1 large Romaine lettuce, chopped into large pieces
- 2 tbsp. chives, chopped to garnish

For Salad Dressing:

- 1/2 tsp. Onion Powder
- 1/2 tsp. Garlic Powder

- 1/2 tbsp. Dijon Mustard

- 1 cup 2% Greek Yogurt

- Kosher Salt and Ground Pepper or to taste

- 1 oz. Anchovy fillets, minced, optional

Instructions

1. In a mixing bowl, add the chicken breasts, then oregano, olive oil, and salt. Coat well with the chicken, cover with plastic and let marinate for at least 1 hour in the fridge.

2. In another bowl, add all the dressing ingredients and mix well until combined and refrigerate.

3. Take the chicken bowl out from the fridge and cool down to room temperature for at least 15 minutes.

4. Heat a large skillet over medium-high heat. Add the marinated chicken and cook for about 6-8 minutes. Flip the chicken and cook for another 4-6 minutes (In between do not move or press the chicken).

5. After it's done, transfer to a cutting board and make slices as you need.

6. In a serving bowl, add the chopped lettuce and avocado, then add peeled and sliced eggs and chicken.

7. Add the prepared dressing to the bowl and toss to coat with the chicken and salad. Add grated parmesan cheese on the top with chopped chives.

8. Add salt and pepper as per taste and enjoy.

18. Keto Grilled Chicken Thighs (Low Carb)

Prep Time: 5 Minutes

Cook Time: 15 Minutes

Servings: 6

Ingredients

- 6 chicken thighs, skinless, boneless
- 2 cloves garlic, minced
- 1 tbsp. of fresh thyme
- 1/4 cup dijon mustard
- 1/4 cup Lakanto Maple Flavored Sugar-Free Syrup
- 2 tbsp. Liquid Aminos or Low Carb Soy Sauce

Instructions

1. Preheat the grill to medium heat.
2. For more flavors, poke little holes over each chicken thighs using a fork to help the chicken soak up the maximum marinade.
3. In a mixing bowl, add thyme, garlic, Lakanto maple syrup, liquid Aminos, and dijon mustard.

4. Place the chicken in a ziplock bag. Pour in the marinade into the ziplock bag and seal. Shake well so that the chicken pieces get evenly coated.

5. Let it sit for about 15 minutes (recommended) or grill right away.

6. Place the marinated chicken on the preheated hot grill.

7. Grill for about 7 minutes on each side or until a meat thermometer reads 165F when inserted into the thickest part of the chicken.

19. Keto Pulled Chicken (Slow Cooker or Instant Pot)

Prep Time: 15 Minutes

Cook Time: 3hrs 2 Minutes

Servings: 8

Ingredients

- 3 pounds chicken breasts, boneless skinless (or chicken thighs, trim off any excess fat)
- 4 ounce butter (or ghee)
- Sauce Ingredients
- 6 ounce tomato paste
- 1/3 cup Swerve Brown sweetener (or Sukrin Gold, Lakanto, or Besti)
- 3 tbsp apple cider vinegar
- 3 tbsp red wine vinegar (if not available add more apple cider vinegar)
- 2 tbsp yellow mustard (i use this one)
- 1 tsp dried thyme
- 1 tsp onion powder
- 1 tsp garlic powder
- 1/8 tsp ground cloves
- 1 tsp black pepper

- 1 tsp salt
- 1/2 tsp celery salt
- 1 tsp liquid smoke

Instructions

1. In a medium bowl, add all the sauce ingredients and combine well.
2. If you are using chicken from the refrigerator, let it cool down to room temperature for about 30 minutes before adding to the pot.
3. Slow Cooker -
4. Place the chicken in a single layer to the crockpot.
5. Add the sauce ingredients evenly all over the chicken.
6. Cover with lid and cook on High for 3-4 hours or Low for 6-8 hours or until the meat thermometer reads 160 F.
7. Remove the chicken, shred the chicken with a mixer or with two forks. Return the chicken to the crockpot, add butter or ghee. Stir, adjust the seasoning as per taste, and serve.

Instant Pot -

1. Add the chicken into the instant pot.

2. Pour the sauce ingredients into the instant pot over the chicken.

3. Lock the lid and close the pressure valve. Cook on high for 5 minutes. When time is up, allow natural pressure release for about 5 minutes before opening the valve.

4. Shred the chicken, add butter and ghee. Stir well and serve with over a salad or with a low carb hamburger.

20. Keto Coconut Chicken (Low Carb Curry)

Prep Time: 20 Minutes

Cook Time: 60 Minutes

Servings: 5

Ingredients

- 5 (about 4-5oz) skinless, boneless chicken thighs (chopped into 1 inch cubes)
- 1/4 red onion, medium, chopped
- 1 cup chicken broth (or bone broth)
- 1 can coconut milk
- 2 1/2 tbsp coconut oil (or ghee/butter)
- 3 cloves garlic, chopped
- 1 tsp ginger, grated
- 1 tbsp curry powder
- 1/2 tsp pink himalayan salt
- 1/2 tsp ground cinnamon

Instructions

1. Heat a skillet or pot over medium-high heat. Add coconut oil or ghee.

2. Add chicken cubes and cook halfway through. Add in chopped onion, garlic, ginger, cinnamon and curry powder. Combine well and cook for about 2-3 minutes.
3. Pour in chicken broth and coconut milk and stir to combine.
4. Reduce heat and simmer for about 40-60 minutes until sauce reaches your desired consistency (If your sauce is not thick enough, cook longer).

DINNER

21. Keto Chicken Fried Rice Cauliflower (Low Carb)

Prep Time: 10 Minutes

Cook Time: 15 Minutes

Servings: 2

Ingredients

- 6 ounces boneless chicken thighs, chopped into small pieces (about 150 g)
- 2 eggs
- 2 large spring onion (about 20 g, white and green part separated)
- 3 cloves garlic, chopped (about 9 g)
- 2 ounces white mushrooms, sliced (about 50 g)
- 2 ounces green peppers (about 50 g)
- 12 ounces cauliflower rice, cooked (about 300 g)
- 1 tablespoon white vinegar
- 1 tablespoon soya sauce
- Salt & pepper
- 2 tablespoon olive oil (you can also use butter or ghee)

Instructions

1. In a bowl beat 2 eggs with little salt and pepper.
2. Heat a wok and add 1 tablespoon of olive oil or butter. Make scrambled egg out of it. Remove from the wok and set aside.
3. Add another tbsp of oil to the wok. Add garlic, spring onion white, and chicken. Add little salt and pepper and fry.
4. Now add in the green peppers and mushrooms and stir until fully cooked.
5. Add the cauliflower rice and the scrambled egg. Mix well.
6. Now add in vinegar and soya sauce and cook for 2-3 minutes.
7. Turn off the heat and add in spring onion greens.

22. Keto Avocado Chicken Salad (Low Carb)

Prep Time: 10 Minutes

Cook Time: 00 Minutes

Servings: 6

Ingredients

- 2 avocados
- 2 cups shredded chicken (or leftover rotisserie chicken)
- ¼ cup red onion, diced (or green onion)
- 1/4 cup mayo
- 2 teaspoons lime juice
- 1 tablespoon fresh coriander leaves (or fresh parsley)
- 1 teaspoon garlic powder
- 1/2 teaspoon salt

Instructions

1. Take a large mixing bowl, add all of the ingredients and mix well until well combined with the avocado.
2. Serve immediately or wrap it with low carb tortillas.

23. Easy Chicken Casserole

Prep Time: 20 Minutes

Cook Time: 50 Minutes

Servings: 6

Ingredients

- 1 (4½ pound) chicken breast/thighs, jointed into 8 pieces
- 150g (5 ounce) button mushrooms
- 2 carrots, cut into chunks
- 100g (4 ounce) streaky bacon, chopped
- 300ml (½ pt) white wine
- 25g (1 ounce) plain flour
- 200g (8 ounce) small onions or shallots, whole and peeled
- 25g (1 ounce) soft butter, plus extra for the sauce
- 1 stick celery, cut into chunks
- Bouquet garni (bay leaf, thyme, parsley stalks, black peppercorns)
- 500ml (18fl ounce) chicken stock
- 2 tablespoon double cream
- Chopped fresh parsley

Instructions

1. In a large frying pan, heat oil and brown the chicken pieces, then transfer to a plate. Now Brown the bacon and put on the plate with the chicken.
2. Before adding the bacon and chicken back into the casserole, add some butter to the oil in the casserole and gently brown the mushrooms and onions.
3. Add the celery, bouquet garni, carrot, chicken stock and wine to the chicken and season well.
4. Cover and cook for 30-40 mins on preheated oven at 170°C.
5. Transfer the vegetables and chicken with a slotted spoon to a large dish and keep warm.
6. To form a paste mix the flour and butter together.
7. Bring the sauce to the boil and add an equal amount of butter and flour mixture (beurre manie) to thicken the sauce, whisking continuously until dissolved. Add the rest of the beurre manie until you have got your desired thickness.
8. Stir in the double cream, then pour over the chicken and garnish with chopped parsley.

24. Blackened Chicken

Prep Time: 5 Minutes

Cook Time: 15 Minutes

Servings: 2

Ingredients

- 1/2 teaspoon paprika
- 1/8 teaspoon salt
- 1/4 teaspoon cayenne pepper
- 1/8 teaspoon onion powder
- 1/8 teaspoon ground white pepper
- 1/4 teaspoon dried thyme
- 1/4 teaspoon ground cumin
- 2 skinless, boneless chicken breast

Instructions

1. Preheat oven to 175 deg. C (350 deg. F). lightly grease a baking sheet. Over high heat for 5 minutes, Heat a cast iron skillet until it is smoking hot.

2. Mix together the cayenne, cumin, paprika, salt, thyme, onion powder and white pepper. Now on both sides, Oil

the chicken breasts with cooking spray, then evenly
with the spice mixture coat the chicken breasts.

3. In the hot pan place your chicken, and cook for 1
   minute. Flip and cook for another 1 minute. On the
   prepared baking sheet, place the breasts.

4. For about 5 minutes bake in the preheated oven until
   the juices run clear and no longer pink in the center.

25. Keto Chinese Chicken and Broccoli (Low Carb)

Prep Time: 10 Minutes

Cook Time: 20 Minutes

Servings: 4

Ingredients

- 1 lb chicken breasts, boneless skinless, cut into strips
- 2 cups broccoli florets, raw
- 1 tablespoon olive oil
- ½ teaspoon sesame oil
- ½ cup liquid aminos (or low carb soy sauce)
- ¼ cup chicken broth
- 3 tablespoon Swerve brown sugar substitute
- 1 teaspoon ginger paste
- 3 teaspoon garlic, minced
- ¼ teaspoon xanthan gum, optional
- 1 tablespoon sesame seeds

Instructions

1. Heat a skillet over medium-high heat. Add sesame and olive oil.

2. Add the chicken, and cook for 3-5 minutes on each side until browned and cooked through. Remove the chicken and set aside.

3. Reduce the heat to medium, add the broccoli florets, place on the lid, and cook until the broccoli is halfway cooked.

4. Add the chicken back to the skillet. Stir well.

5. In a mixing bowl, add the brown sugar substitute, soy sauce, chicken broth, minced garlic, and garlic paste. Combine well.

6. Pour the sauce mixture into the skillet over the chicken and broccoli. Toss to coat.

7. Add xanthan gum to thicken the sauce as per your liking. Add a little at a time. Add more liquid if it's too thick.

8. Let it cook for a few more minutes or until the chicken and broccoli have soaked enough sauce flavors. Sprinkle with sesame seeds.

26. Keto Balsamic Caprese Chicken (Low Carb)

Prep Time: 5 Minutes

Cook Time: 30 Minutes

Servings: 5

Ingredients

- 2 teaspoons Italian seasoning
- 4 chicken breasts, boneless, skinless
- 1 teaspoon black pepper
- 1 teaspoon salt and pepper
- 2 tablespoons butter, divided
- 1/2 cup chicken broth or cooking wine
- 2 cups cherry tomatoes, sliced
- 1 tablespoon balsamic vinegar + more for drizzling
- 4 ounces fresh mozzarella cheese
- 1/4 cup fresh basil

Instructions

1. Preheat oven to 350 degrees F.
2. In a medium bowl, place the chicken and season with Italian seasoning, salt and pepper.

3. Heat up a large skillet over medium heat. Add 1 tablespoon butter, once melted, add the seasoned chicken and cook for about 2-3 minutes on each side.

4. Remove the chicken from the skillet and set aside

5. Add the chicken broth to deglaze the pan. Scrape up any brown bits from the bottom of the pan and bring the broth to a simmer.

6. Cook for about 5-6 minutes until reduced by half. Stir in the remaining tablespoon of butter and balsamic glaze.

7. Add the chicken back to the pan, and fully coat with balsamic glaze. Add in the cherry tomatoes and top the chicken with the fresh mozzarella.

8. Place the skillet in the oven and bake for about 20 minutes or until the internal temperature of the chicken has reached 165 degrees F when checked with the meat thermometer.

9. Top with additional balsamic glaze and fresh basil.

27. Keto Slow Cooker Ranch Chicken (Low Carb)

Prep Time: 5 Minutes

Cook Time: 8hrs 3 Minutes

Servings: 6

Ingredients

- 1 1/2 pounds chicken breast, boneless, skinless
- 1 tablespoon butter, unsalted
- 4 ounces cream cheese
- 1 (1 ounce) package of seasoning mix by Hidden Valley Ranch
- 8-10 jarred pepperoncini peppers

Instructions

1. Add all the ingredients in a 2-quart slow cooker
2. Cook on low for 8 hours.
3. Shred the chicken by using two forks and put it back to the pot. Stir well and adjust the seasoning as per the taste.

28. Baked Chicken

Prep Time: 15 Minutes

Cook Time: 45 Minutes

Servings: 4

Ingredients

- 1 teaspoon seasoning salt
- 4 boneless skinless chicken breasts
- 1/2 cup freshly grated Parmesan cheese
- 1/2 teaspoon ground black pepper
- 1 teaspoon garlic powder
- 1 container (5 ounces) plain Greek Yogurt

Instructions

1. Prchcat oven to 375° F.
2. With the non-stick cooking spray, spray the baking dish.
3. Combine Parmesan cheese, yogurt, and seasonings.
4. Spread over chicken breasts. Bake until chicken is cooked through and no longer pink from inside for

about 45 minutes, and topping is browned. Serve immediately.

29. Chicken Marsala

Prep Time: 10 Minutes

Cook Time: 20 Minutes

Servings: 4

Ingredients

- 1/4 cup all-purpose flour for coating
- 1/2 teaspoon salt
- 1/4 teaspoon ground black pepper
- 1/2 teaspoon dried oregano
- 4 skinless, boneless chicken breast halves - pounded 1/4 inch thick
- 4 tablespoons butter
- 4 tablespoons olive oil
- 1 cup sliced mushrooms
- 1/2 cup Marsala wine
- 1/4 cup cooking sherry

Instructions

1. In a bowl, mix together the salt, pepper flour and oregano. Coat chicken pieces in flour mixture.

2. Over medium heat melt butter in oil (in a large skillet).

3. Place chicken in the pan and cook, until lightly brown. Turn over chicken pieces, and add mushrooms. Pour in sherry & wine. Cover skillet cook chicken for 10 minutes until no longer pink in the center and juices run clear.

30. Chicken Stew

Prep Time: 20 Minutes

Cook Time: 2hrs 2 Minutes

Servings: 6

Ingredients

- 1 pound chicken tenders
- 4 cups water
- 2 stalks celery, cut into chunks
- 1 sweet potato, diced
- 2 potatoes, diced
- 1 (8 ounce) can tomato sauce
- 1 (15 ounce) can peas
- 1 cup cooked rice
- 2 bay leaves
- 3 carrots, cut into chunks

Instructions

1. Stir water, celery, potatoes, chicken, carrots, peas, tomato sauce, sweet potato, and bay leaves together in a pot.

2. Cook at a simmer, on medium heat for 1 hour 45 minutes.

3. Into the soup stir cooked rice and cook for 15 minutes until the rice separates into grains and are hot.